Be Limit*less*:

Trusting God's Plan

Kizzy McCray-Sheppard

Be Limitless:
Trusting God's Plan

Copyright © 2021 by Kizzy McCray-Sheppard

(ISBN 978-1-7375310-5-0)

All rights reserved. No part of this book may be reproduced or transmitted in any form or by any means without written permission from the author.

Disclaimer: The following versions of the Bible may have been referenced: New International Version (NIV), King James Version (KJV), New Living Translation (NLT), English Standard Version (ESV), New King James (NKJV), New International Reader's Version (NIRV), Christian Standard Bible (CSB), Common English Bible (CEB), The Message (MSG)

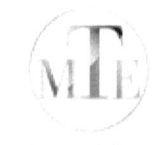

MTE Publishing
mtepublishing.com

Acknowledgments

The publication of this literary work would not be possible without God. He is the source of my limitless mindset and lifestyle. So, I dedicate this work to Him, first.

To my husband Robert, thank you for your consistent support, love, and patience. You've helped me embrace Limitless Possibilities Now™. You always lift me up, and you've never made me feel like I had to minimize myself *with* you. I love you and I am eternally grateful.

To my son Zephaniah, you are truly a miracle from God. You are very kind and caring towards all people. I am blessed to be your mother; and I know your greatness is limitless!

To Nakia, you are an irreplaceable gift from God, and I am so grateful for you! You're strong, beautiful, and loving. I admire your dedication to the things of God. You will accomplish every goal you set, because there are no limits to what YOU can do *with* God.

Zephaniah and Nakia, I pray that I embody limitlessness before you every day. Never lose sight of who God created you to be.

To my mother, Catherine, you have always been my personal cheerleader! You are a treasure from God, and I am blessed to be your daughter. You epitomize what it means to LOVE limitlessly!

To my daddy, the first man to love me unconditionally… I miss you more and more daily, and I cherish our memories. I dedicate this book to you. I know you're smiling on me from Heaven saying, "Look at my baby girl!"

Finally, to my extended family, friends, colleagues, and associates, this book is for you. Let's manifest and seize life's Limitless Possibilities Now ™!

Foreword

By Shawn Fair, CEO and Founder of the Leadership Experience Tour

As an individual who has never ascribed to mediocrity, I recognize opportune situations and individuals who grasp and create opportunities! Kizzy McCray-Sheppard, the *Limitless Thought Leader*™ is intelligent, driven, and determined. I met her at one of my Leadership Experience Tours for aspiring speakers. Mrs. Sheppard didn't possess the spotlight, but she created space that allowed her to share the spotlight with others! This is a sign of a true leader. Consequently, I reached out to her because I was drawn to her ability to make impactful connections.

Kizzy epitomizes what it is to be limitless. The stories behind her triumphs and tragedies, allow others to understand her innate ability to progress beyond circumstantial limitations.

Her debut literary work, "Be Limitless: Trusting God's Plan," encourages her readers to fully embrace the mentality of being limitless! Kizzy understands that anything is achievable, obstacles are conquerable, and when God is the center of our drive it makes us unstoppable!

Table of Contents

Acknowledgments iii

Foreword vi

Introduction: Repurposed x

Chapters

1. The Ladder and the Bridge 1

2. Marriage is a Covenant, not a Contract 8

3. The Limitless Cs of Relationships 15

4. Limitless Faith 22

5. Rebirth: Another Chance to be Limitless 27

6. Processing Loss 35

7. Just Beat It: Anxiety 41

8. Purposed for It 50

9. The Limitless Formula.......................................57

About the Author 68

Introduction

Repurposed

During my childhood and my early adult years, I thought I'd either be a doctor or a lawyer. I have always been passionate about taking care of people and talking- A LOT. In fact, my brother always called me little Miss Chatterbox.

November 16, 1994, I was in 10th-grade and my mom left to visit my uncle's. The accident happened about five miles away from our home in Bronson, FL. Darkness loomed across the distance and the busyness of the day had slowed down. There were no streetlights, and a cast iron trailer was left parked halfway on the street. My uncle's tan Toyota Celica plowed directly into it. Mom was in the passenger seat and as a result of the impact, the motor landed in her lap and crushed several of her bones instantly.

When I arrived at the scene, I could hear my mother screaming. I tried my best to get to her, but my family members restrained me as I screamed, "Noooooo, I want to see my momma, please!" My sobs and pleas were unanswered. I was distraught, I felt like I was going to lose my momma. They had to cut her out of the car. She had 10 broken ribs, a broken pelvis, and a concussion. My uncle was fine, but my mother was on the verge of death.

When we arrived at the hospital, they rushed her behind closed doors. I was with my mom every single day for a year and attended every appointment with her. That's what led me into the medical field. That's when I started saying I wanted to become a doctor. In my senior year, I said I wanted to become a nurse. God allowed me to walk out my mom's dreams because she desired to be a nurse.

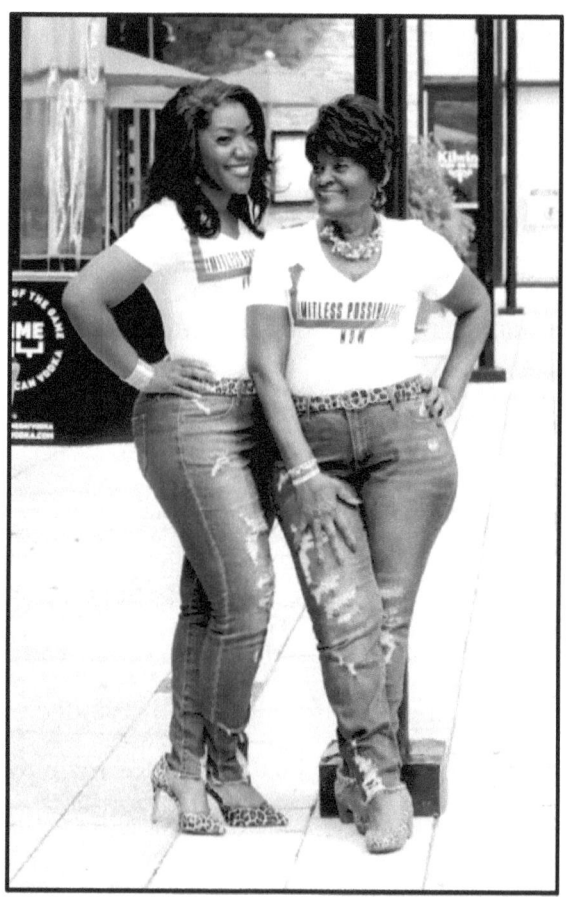

Me with my precious mother, Catherine Smith.

My mom grew up in rural Georgia and picked cotton. She picked over 200 pounds of cotton a day after school. My mom didn't achieve her dreams because she put her family's needs first. It was natural for me to pick up the baton and pursue our dream for the better. That's what we're supposed to do [be better than our parents and make them proud]. Mom only went as far as a nurse's aide. She also did private sitting for an elderly couple. After mom's clients passed, and my brother and I got older, momma returned to work at the school board as a lunchroom server and custodian. Nevertheless, she lit a flame on the inside of me that led me into my destiny.

Chapter 1

The Ladder and the Bridge

I've always been a person who helped people. When I was in first grade, I befriended a boy named Roger, who was non-verbal. He was white and had sandy blonde hair with brown eyes. I spent lots of time with him. I loved him like a brother. Unfortunately, Roger and his family relocated, and I was completely heartbroken. This is how I learned to love and have compassion for all people. Great nurses exude this; however, some of us are called to this profession while others just choose it. For those of us who are called, we love and care for our patients while they are in our care then we release them. The job description is engraved on our heart; therefore, the work is ministry.

I attended college with one of my high school friends. Immediately, we met new people and started making friends. Then I met a peculiar young lady. We'd go to pick up food and I remember driving into a local restaurant and ordering. My roommate ordered her food, and I noticed the young lady we befriended didn't order. So, I ordered two of everything and when we returned to the dorm, I split the drink and we ate together like a family. From that moment on, we looked out for each other.

I must credit my seemingly innate altruism to my grandmother and mother. They fed perfect strangers and helped folks get jobs throughout the Levy County area. I was raised around women who extended a helping hand often, therefore, helping others has always been effortless for me.

I remember one of my brother's classmates was down on his luck. My mom sent my brother to find him to ensure he had warm shelter. This is the Hannah way [love people without question].

By nature, I'm a helper. I've always been a ladder and bridge, even to those who attempted to burn them down. Nevertheless, I have trusted God's plan and He led me to great success. However, success isn't success without being a ladder or a bridge to others.

In 1999, I enlisted in the United States Air Force. My mom's older sister passed away from cancer. She taught me how to cook along with my grandmother and mom. When my mom had the accident, my aunt helped me take care of her. I spent a lot of time with my beloved aunt. When she passed, it awakened what was already inside of me [my call to the medical field].

I looked for a way to take care of myself and earn a degree. My parents didn't want me to go, but I knew what I needed to do. My mom let me go at the will of my aunt who passed. I was homesick but it was the best decision I ever made. I was a medic and worked at the Flight Medicine Clinic where I took care of the high-ranking generals and pilots.

I rose through the ranks, and I was promoted six months sooner than my peers. I received the Air Force Commendation Medal for Heroism. I was off duty and witnessed this older lady hit the tail end of a truck that flipped over. I went to the aid of a young man. I eventually found out his dad was a high-ranking chief. I just happened to be in the right place at the right time. I had an emergency kit in my car ready to spring into action. I stopped traffic to cross the street, climbed into the truck [that was on its side] with him, and reminded him to remain calm. I could tell he had a head injury because he had fluid coming from his ears. I stabilized his neck until paramedics arrived.

A year later, I went to medical records at Scott Air Force Base. This day was particularly different. I met a young lady, who eventually became my soul sister. She and her husband were eagerly awaiting the birth of their second child. When she gave birth to their daughter, she had a head full of hair. I was one proud auntie [and still am some 20-plus years later]. During one of our many conversations, we discussed life after the military. I encouraged her to go to school. I knew a college education would help her provide for her family. However, she felt quite uncertain. So, I told her the military provides educational benefits for service men and women to earn a degree.

When she enrolled, I kept her babies while she completed her studies. Her education gave her the foundation she needed for a successful life. Thankfully, as I blessed her, God blessed me. Life requires give and take. However, we must give more than we take. We should be genuinely excited to witness the wins of others and vice versa. When we're either a bridge or a ladder for someone else, it sets us up for limitless possibilities!

I served nine years in the service [four years active duty and five years in the Air National Guard]. All the while, I knew my steps were ordered by God. Therefore, He allowed me to understand the benefit of sowing into others consistently. My harvest was bound to be plentiful and abundant… no matter what happened later. I had to learn to trust God's plan.

Lesson: Ladders and bridges are tools that connect people, places, and things— BE BOTH… because you never know when you will need to climb or cross one to reach your destiny.

Chapter 2

Marriage is a Covenant, not a Contract

In 2001, I got married. I approached the union as if it was a contract and not a covenant. There were lots of deal breakers and lots of loopholes. I had already pinpointed them going into the marriage. Additionally, I knew I wasn't supposed to get married because I had doubts.

I remember calling people because I was nervous at the onset. They passed it off as cold feet. However, there was one friend who said, "Don't do it." I spoke with my mom, and she thought that we should wait but wanted us to be happy. That's when I learned when you get married you don't have cold feet. If it's something God ordained, you will know it. It was something we put together— not God. He fit what I thought I needed in a man... He made the cut. He didn't have children and he had a career. He had to be tall, dark, and handsome [although he was only dark and handsome]. We were different so much so that the relationship crumbled after only two years. We were young and needed God. However, we didn't realize just how much we needed Him in our hearts and in our marriage.

Remember, we can make our best attempt to build a man, but he won't be who God built and customized him to be [if we do it]. My second husband is the one the Lord sent. While he isn't tall and dark; he sure is handsome. I met him eight miles from where I grew up. I never knew him, but we knew the same people. We met at a cookout and my cousin, and her husband wanted me to meet him. When we met, I immediately knew he wasn't my type and besides, I didn't want anyone from the area. Nevertheless, I said to myself nah, he doesn't fit the bill. Then he went on to say that I was his wife and that I was the woman of his dreams. I literally thought he was crazy and laughed at him. He responded, "I actually had a dream about you, and you are going to be my wife." Ultimately, we were friends, and my sole purpose was to lead him to Christ (nothing more, nothing less).

He's what God wanted for me; although, I didn't want to accept it because I was still wrestling with him not being "my type". He already had a child —strike one— so being serious with him was off the table. Nevertheless, when we met, he was a "special occasion" churchgoer. He only went to church on Easter, Mother's Day, and Christmas.

As we cultivated our relationship, he followed me to church. My mission was simple, I wanted him to fall in love with God for himself. I even encouraged him to date other people. I picked up and moved away to Savannah, GA. He continued to call and see my family. In fact, my mother called him son. Years prior to marriage, we were intimate. However, when God reconnected us, three years, later we rekindled our courtship. We both knew what we needed to do to have a Godly marriage. Therefore, he respected my mind, body and soul, and he only kissed my forehead until the day we tied the knot.

In 2009, I attended the fireman's ball for Christmas. He was sitting at a table with some guests. I was ready to leave and although we didn't attend the event together, I walked over and said, "Let's go." He did just that and we left.

I remember it like it was yesterday, our church went on a corporate fast [with prayer]. He said the Lord answered his prayer. He announced on Celebration Sunday [the Sunday before the Superbowl] that we were getting married [without a ring]. I said to myself, "He is announcing this to the church without an official proposal." I'm a woman of order and strongly believe everything, particularly a proposal [to me], should be done in an orderly fashion [with a touch of fanfare]. And although this was not typical for me, it felt so right.

As we get older, we see things differently. A man who loves God was at the top of my list. We started with a friendship, and we *communicated*. The prophecy was fulfilled, when I became his wife on October 14, 2011. The theme for our wedding was a *covenant* promise. He didn't fit my idea of "Mr. Right"; nevertheless, he is God's choice for me. I still believe he's always been head over heels for me from the start. There haven't been any *conflicts* that weren't easily resolved.

Today, we encourage those considering marriage and married couples through a marriage ministry called, *A Covenant Promise*.

Marriage is a covenant not a contract. A covenant is a promise and an agreement between two individuals and *God*. Just like God made a covenant with His children, He has the same intent for marriage. Now a contract is a written agreement between two parties that's legally binding but there are loopholes and potential breeches. This happens when one party fails to perform and/or deliver. Some go into marriage with a contractual mindset and not a covenant mindset. When marriage becomes a record of "tit for tat" the marriage will be irrefutably shallow. Covenant realizes the relationship isn't perfect [it never will be]. However, marriages that are ordained by God are perfected by His promises. Covenant requires trusting God's plan [keeping

God as the head] and a contract is about deliverables man's way. Conflicts arise when deliverables [expectations] aren't met within a certain timeframe. Additionally, it removes grace and mercy from the equation. God is the equation, there are no rectifiable solutions without Him!

Lesson: Covenant marriages are full of grace and endowed with the blessings of God. Contracts are full of legalese and loopholes. Allow love to win and refuse to keep score… Marriage is a covenant, not a contract.

Chapter 3

The Limitless Cs of Relationships

The establishment of any relationship requires individuals to consciously evaluate the purpose of their connection. Biblically, Christ has provided the foundation for all relationships which is unconditional love because it is sacrificial. When our relationships are rooted in love, the commitment transitions from selfish to selfless. This is the sacrifice of love... when two become one, everything is felt mutually; sickness and health, poverty, and wealth, and hurt and healing.

I've learned that there are limitless qualities inside of each of us, and when applied to other areas in our lives, we begin to live limitless. Even in relationships that we build through marriage, work, friendships and through acquaintances— a limitless life awaits. God stretches us to the limit so that we can live limitlessly. While most people will never admit this, I learned to love my husband unconditionally *after* we married. That's where the growth happens, during the journey. This is also how we acquired limitless possibilities within our marriage. We were divinely *connected* as friends, first, and then lovers. I believe God intended it to be that way because of the mountains we'd have to *conquer*. Marriage is about friendship; it is the foundation.

One night as we slept our hands intertwined, this wasn't intentional, but it was divinely orchestrated. Both my husband and I were kind of freaked out because neither of us remembered reaching for each other's hands. We believed this was God's way of revealing to us that

He was our matchmaker, and whatever God has joined no man or thing can tear apart.

We've surmounted several mountains, but our greatest mountain was dealing with my own independence. I set myself up for success by making the right *choices*. I didn't need a man to define me or take care of me. I knew my own strength; therefore, I had to allow my husband to lead. The greatest weapons were my mindset and my mouth. I didn't need a man, but I wanted one. I had to learn to use my words wisely. My independence is something I built, and I wasn't going to allow anyone to tear it down [but me]. My husband knew I was independent, and he didn't need me to yell it from the mountaintop. Interestingly enough, I knew I had a good husband and I refused to allow anyone to inch up on him and destroy what we had.

Although, I hammered at it with my own independence and *crushed* him with my words, but like God, he loved me still...so much so that he shared a scripture with me that would shift my perspective: Proverbs: 14:1 *The wise woman builds her house but with her own hands the foolish one tears hers down.* Eventually, I figured out that I needed to become the wise woman and build my house, so I tamed my tongue and humbly applauded my independence. I never said, "I can take care of myself...I was taking care of myself before you!" I buried those words and never resurrected them again.

Women of color are taught that we must be *strong*. Unfortunately, it is our "strength" that won't allow us to be vulnerable enough to say, "I don't need you to save me; however, I desire for you to care for me, value me, respect me and love me...I want you to make me feel safe [while honoring my independence]." Furthermore, women of color believe we must be tough like our grandmothers/ancestors without realizing we don't have to be. God places the right people [soulmates] in our lives to help us gracefully relinquish our independence as a badge of honor. Understand that we often fight throughout our lives and when God says to release it [and we obey], the fight *ceases*.

Another mountain we had to surmount was the art of building good *communication* skills. Once my husband decided he would buy a motorcycle without talking to me about it. While some people call it a "mid-life crisis," I called it disrespectful. It was an investment that *we* needed to discuss and plan out. Halfway *communicating* is not communicating and will cause things to crash and burn, quickly. When he got home, he said, "God blessed me with it." He went on bragging about how it was a limited, anniversary edition and it only had one previous owner who just so happened to be a pastor. He had already gotten his motorcycle [a Harley] license and had informed a friend that he was getting one. Honestly speaking, looking back it was nothing more than deception. I threw it in his face every opportunity I got for years. I had a mental list of wrongs and kept score until God *convicted* me. My husband apologized and I did too.

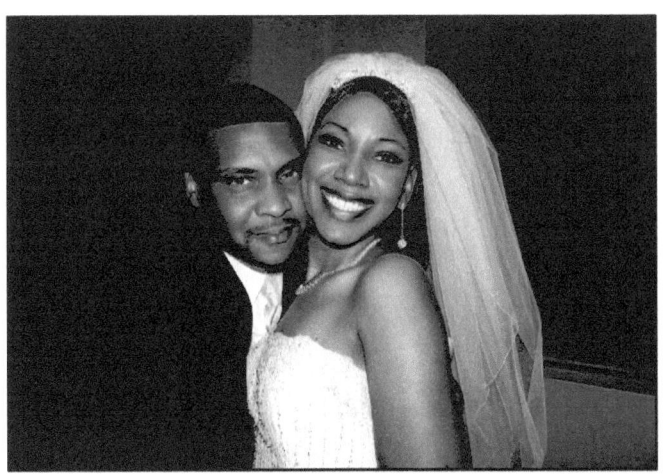

My husband Robert and me on our wedding day.

On another occasion, we passed a mansion and I told him that I wanted it. He seemed unmoved. I said to him, "You have a limited mindset. God never allowed me to be content, because it leads to complacency. He has so much more for us and will exceed our wildest expectations, if we don't put limits on Him." After this, a lightbulb went off, and we fully understood the limitless principles of being on one accord.

Lesson: Communicate often and openly about everything because communication is key for building trust and respect in marriage. As a result, we now have a limitless marriage, and you can too!

Chapter 4

Limitless Faith

God strategically put us in places and positions, although we don't know His intentions. The setup is divinely planned so we fulfill our purpose. Therefore, we must trust God's plan in every assignment. Naturally, we want to see it before we believe it.

Unfortunately, when we decide that seeing is believing, we usually cannot see beyond our current circumstances. Then we forfeit the faith that is required to make it through. This frustrates our faith, which is the prerequisite to tapping into our ability to be limitless. Undoubtedly, it is difficult to trust in God when we feel as though we are being buried alive by our reality. However, we must *always* consider God's track record. His layout for our lives is not just perfect but it intentionally makes us benefactors of His blessings.

In 2013, I resigned from UF Health where I was a critical care nurse. I accepted a position at the VA, as a staff nurse within Hospice and Palliative care. However, in a little more than a month's time, I was promoted to a leadership position as an assistant nurse manager. While in the position, I was able to impact many lives beyond patient care. I mentored three CNAs who eventually became registered nurses. I also mentored LPNs who are RNs, today. This was a part of my divine assignment. My supervisor and I were lifelines and support systems for aspiring nurses. I volunteered to watch their kids while they went back to school to earn their degrees.

I did what I was supposed to do while I was *assigned* there. I helped a total of seven nurses become limitless. When the last mentee completed her nursing program, my assignment was completed as well. It was time for me to continue my pursuit to become a limitless nurse practitioner. I took a part-time position and never looked back.

Before I left the chief nurse asked, "Are you sure you want to leave all this money?" I responded quite casually and said, "Sometimes you have to go down to come up." I had no clue the level of faith I'd need to go as far down as I went. Every time I thought I had reached the bottom; I was made to go a little bit deeper. The more I trusted God, the more He tested my faith in Him. I didn't just understand but I came to know that God's provision will irrefutably sustain us. I wasn't just "faith-talking," I became a faith-filled believer of God's limitless love for us!

It is impossible to live off $434 bi-weekly, but my husband and I made it because God gave us a "two fish and five loaves" type of miracle until it was no longer needed. My husband covered 90 percent of our bills that exceeded $5,000 a month. I would plan meals to make sure food stretched, we had nothing to waste. Best of all, we didn't lose anything, particularly our faith.

I had to go even deeper when it was time to graduate and remit fees for certification and licensing. My faith was tested all the way to the end. I flew to Chicago (twice) to complete my program. Nevertheless, in July, my family flew to Chicago for my graduation from the nurse practitioner's program. By God's grace, I completed the program and maintained a high level of academic excellence!

During this process, I was broken, shaped, strengthened, separated, restored, purified, and elevated. The ultimate outcome is total victory! We come out thinking differently, believing differently and knowing God differently. This makes trusting the plan worth it!

Lesson: Faith is the prerequisite to be and become limitless because God's plans for our lives are manifested through the work we do faithfully.

Chapter 5

Rebirth: Another Chance to be Limitless

March 2020, at the onset of COVID-19, my life changed. In October of 2019, I applied for a few positions. I didn't put much thought into it because I knew I would be at the VA. Surprisingly; I got a call from a recruiter for a position that I did not directly apply for. I left the interview knowing I landed the job.

As I drove down the road, I saw a bus with a sign for Community Hospice and Palliative Care. This was a sign. The company is built on community values, with a mission to improve the quality of life for patients and families. It was founded by a pastor and two nurses more than 42 years ago.

God is intentional regarding every aspect of our lives. January 3, 2020, I left my position at the VA Hospital after more than 10 years of federal service. Nevertheless, I was in the right place at the right time when my life flashed before my eyes. Friday, March 27, 2020, I almost died! However, that day God reminded me that He is a miracle worker.

I was traveling with my Community Hospice team, then COVID-19 happened.

The world changed as we knew it. I had to manage extra caseloads. That day I had an afternoon meeting. As I prepared to leave my house, our daughter called saying, "My car has broken down." My husband went to meet her and wait for the tow truck then returned home. While driving to my office, I listened to the song: *This Week* by Anthony Brown & Group Therapy. As I turned into the office parking lot, I felt a paralyzing pain; it was the worst pain I'd ever felt. The pain was worse than labor pains. I got out of my car, and I felt a heaviness fall on me as I walked into the office. I was sweating profusely. I made it to the door, and it took all the energy I had to open it.

Finally, I made it into the office, and I fell to my knees immediately. I called out to my colleagues for help. Billie rushed to my aid and yelled out for the others in the office, "Bring the prayer blanket and pillow from my office!" They immediately checked my vitals. There was so much happening around me at that moment. EMS picked me up and rushed me to UF Health. They took me into a room. I heard several questions, but I didn't have the capacity to speak. I was foaming out of my mouth and my speech was slurred. I conducted a wellness check in my head based on what I was experiencing. I thought I was having a stroke, but how could that be? I didn't have hypertension, pre-existing health conditions or any illnesses that were comorbidities. I was in excellent health!

Although it was the onset of the global pandemic, the medical staff allowed my husband to come in the back. A doctor came in and scanned me. He turned to my husband and said, "She has a stomach full of fluid...OH! Do you see the baby in her uterus?!" Then I heard the other doctor say, "We have to move now! We must save her life!" They inserted IV lines and I needed two units of blood STAT [a medical term for move NOW]!

God placed an angel in the ER, a male nurse with an angelic voice. He started singing, *Nothing but the blood of Jesus*. This was the first indication that God was with me. The following morning I found out that I had lost three liters of blood and my blood pressure was fatally low at 50/30. Women only have 4.5-5 liters of blood in our bodies, and I lost more than half. I should have died—but God! They replaced two units of blood in the ER, to stabilize me for surgery. If I hadn't received a blood transfusion, I wouldn't have made it.

My body did everything it could to fight, as my life slowly attempted to fade away. If I didn't know how to do anything else, I knew how to pray! If only I called on the powerful name of Jesus, I knew He would answer me!

During this life-altering moment, I realized that I was the miracle that I had sung about less than 24 hours prior. We don't often get "do-overs" in life, it is completely uncommon. However, God granted me another chance, and now I celebrate two birthdays. The first on October 18th and the second on March 27th!

On my second birthday, I lost two babies (one in my tubes, the other in my uterus) but God spared me. Their lives were sacrificed so I could complete the good work He already started.

After my brush with death, I stopped procrastinating [regarding everything] and most importantly, I made myself a priority. I ditched the notion of needing anyone's approval or validation. I no longer waited for opportunities to come my way, I created them and purposefully sought them out.

Now, I do everything that God purposed for me to do in *my* lifetime! This time around, I'm all in… and nothing can or will derail the plans that God has for my life [or yours]! I will not leave anyone behind who needs my guidance. This is how I live a life that is purpose-filled while fulfilling my purpose and God's plan. My life is a testament of the limitless opportunities I have to ensure the upbuilding of His kingdom. I will plant seeds and speak life into every person I come in contact with, while reminding them of their God-given greatness.

Again, March 27th, 2020, was all a part of God's plan. My assignment at Community Hospice was the manifestation of Jeremiah 29:11. As I was rushed out of the office, the sincere prayers of my coworkers commanded God to respond. I've never had colleagues not only pray for me, but they genuinely cared about my family as well. My colleagues stayed in contact with my husband throughout my recovery. They made sure my family had meals and they assisted us in every way they could. I felt like I was a beloved relative within their immediate family. I cannot begin to articulate how much their love has proven how much God loves me. He is strategic in everything, and this causes us to be limitless!

Lesson: I have come to understand that it is in our weakest moments that God performs his GREATEST miracles. His strength is perfect when our weaknesses seem to consume us. God is intentional in everything regarding us; even when it seems our chances to live out His will are limited. God is the God of another chance!

Chapter 6

Processing Loss

As I processed the unbearable grief, I couldn't help but reflect on the words of our son, Zephaniah, who said, I would be having two babies. I was conflicted. I couldn't imagine my family without me as I imagined our family with twins. My husband reaffirmed me and encouraged me, which gave me *some* hope. I was thankful that God had given him comforting words of faith that would lead us to our expected end (Jeremiah 29:11). He lovingly expressed, "I can't imagine doing life without you, I will choose you every time over having another child, you are irreplaceable. God can always bless us in another way!"

As the days went by, I knew my son and husband needed me. God always gives our hearts a reason to go on. I found the strength to grieve the losses while communicating with close family members. Now I know why women in the bible who couldn't bear children felt ashamed because that's what I felt...shameful and inadequate. Why could I have one child but not three? I had to process so many different emotions. Nevertheless, I realized the quickest way to gain hope was to count my blessings. I thanked God for the one child that I was blessed to birth. I also thanked God for the daughter I was blessed with through marriage. I also thanked Him for my godchildren (all 10 of them), and for my nieces and nephews. Most importantly, I was thankful that God spared my life so that I could still be here to be a wife and mom.

As I continued to count my blessings, I processed the emotions of grief. I couldn't escape the thoughts of being a mom to twins. We were so elated and overjoyed that God had decided to bless us with another opportunity to be the parents of another little person, especially after having a previous miscarriage that left a hole in our hearts. Interestingly enough, God had given our son Zephaniah insight to know something was different. He walked over to me and placed his head on my stomach and said, "Mommy you're pregnant and there are two of them." Robert and I looked at each other strangely because we couldn't believe our little prophet had spoken such a thing.

At that point, we thought what if God gave us double for our trouble and we actually had twins. We started to come up with names and imagined what it would be like to hear extra little feet running around our home. My imagination ran wild with thoughts of a beautiful brown curly-haired girl! Then I immediately realized, I would have to learn how to do hair—YIKES! I could see her hair styled in puffs and pink bows! Oh how I would enjoy dressing her up... and besides, girls have the best clothes. We would dress in mommy and me outfits; she would be a mini Kizzy...just a prissy little thing! I could see her nursery full of angels and fairies, pink and gold everywhere.

If we had a little boy, he would be just as dapper as his daddy. The classic look would definitely fit him, suspenders, paperboy hats and fedoras. He would be ready to grace the cover of Baby GQ. We were so ready for our home to be filled with coos and smiles. We had begun to imagine how excited Zephaniah would be to finally be a big brother... he had been asking for a baby brother or sister since he was four.

We believed this was the perfect time because he would be such a great helper. It was a time for new beginnings and God was now opening a new door to parenthood for us once again. Everything seemed so right, as we believed it was God's perfect timing.

However, our dreams were shattered, and the nightmare of another miscarriage became our reality. I didn't understand why God allowed me to get pregnant then lose not one, but *two* babies? The loss of material things is difficult, and I've had my share of losses.

Purposely, when a woman has an embryo inside of her, it is a soul tie. The bond of a mother's love causes her to unselfishly care about her unborn child before she ever physically has the chance to hold him or her. It wasn't fair and I didn't believe this tragic loss could have been a *godly* act. I felt forsaken, and I questioned the sovereignty of God because I needed answers.

Grief numbs us and it allows us to feel everything simultaneously. I had no choice… I had to process every stage- from the initial shock, depression, and anger- to the blame, regret, and shame. These stages helped me to gain a greater sense of gratitude. To attain this perspective, I prayed, meditated, received support, and committed to counseling. I refused to merely exist, and I chose to live again, one moment at a time.

Lesson: If you're experiencing loss, my prayer for you is anchored in Matthew 5:4, which reads, *Blessed are those who mourn because they will be comforted.* Even loss plays an essential part in our process of becoming limitless.

Chapter 7

Just Beat It: Anxiety

Have you ever felt trapped in an alternate world? One that you created in your mind. It feels like you are being suffocated by your thoughts (with your thoughts). All too often, this is a reality that many people are unwilling to deal with and discuss, particularly in the Black community.

It was November 4, 2002, and I was awakened from what I believed was a nightmare. However, the events of the nightmare manifested a few months later. I had a dream that my daddy had gotten fatally ill and was eventually hospitalized, then died. The premonition within my dream revealed everything... even the funeral. I'm a dreamer and I've finally become confident in the truthfulness of them. My dreams have the capability to send me into a joyful praise or vehement sobbing.

During this time I was living in Illinois, so I picked up the phone and called my mother. I could not keep what I had dreamt from her. When I told momma about the dream she said, "Your dad is OK, I spoke with him a few days ago… your dream was *just a dream*." After our conversation, I still didn't feel assured so I called my daddy. He also insisted that he was good. Then he said, "Daddy's fine. I've just been having a little back pain from the fall I had a while back. Michelle, it was just a dream, I'm OK!" However, I knew in my heart that something wasn't right. I just couldn't shake the dread and heaviness I felt. My dream haunted me for three months until I received *the call*.

On January 25, 2003, we found out my daddy was fatally ill as a result of medical negligence. My dad had critical hypoglycemia (blood sugar less than 54) and his glucose level was dangerously low at the time of his death. A normal blood glucose level for someone with type II diabetes (that is controlled with medication) should be 80-130.

My world changed after my father's death. I was truly daddy's little girl. I was his baby, and everyone knew it! He was the first man to tell me he loved me, he taught me how to ride a bike, and showed me how I should be treated and loved by a man. He was my real-life superhero. I never thought I would be in my twenties, facing one of the hardest days of my life. International Lovers' day (Valentine's Day) had just passed, and on February 15, 2003, I said my goodbyes to my daddy. If I never celebrated Valentine's Day again,

I would be OK… Besides, I couldn't because the date was too close to daddy's death. He wasn't supposed to leave so soon, he was supposed to be here when I had children. I had always pictured my dad being a playful and cheerful grandfather, who would take my children to UF's Homecoming parade, FAMU's Battle of the Bands, and the Florida Classic. My dad did all of these things with me during my childhood and adolescent years. Unfortunately, life didn't work out this way, and I had to accept the fact that my daddy was never coming back.

A year later, I rededicated my life to Christ. I needed Him… I came to truly understand and experience how God is a Father to the fatherless.

As grief settled in, so did fear, anxiety and depression. I relived that moment in my mind over and over again, until it led to further darkness. In my mind, I saw my mother's house catching on fire and me not being there to save her. There was not a true threat of this happening, except in my mind, and I had dreamt it! I suffered from severe insomnia. I had dreams about my dad, and I'd wake up crying uncontrollably; and I endured the unnerving effects of PTSD for almost five years.

My mother used to have a Morning Tru Gas tank outside of the home to heat our house and light the oven. She had not used it in years, because everything in the house was upgraded to electric. In a vision I had, the gas tank caused an explosion. I immediately called my mother and told her that we needed to have the tank removed. After unexpectedly losing my dad, I seriously thought that if I were not home, then I would lose my mother, too. The thought alone caused my anxiety to intensify. My heart would race, and I felt as if I couldn't breathe. I chose to ignore the symptoms; however, my mom would pray for me. She also instructed me to plant Psalm 91 in my heart, and I did, but my faith wasn't strong enough to crush my fears. Each year I experienced another setback, especially during the holidays and daddy's birthday.

I recently started celebrating Valentine's Day a couple of years ago, because I understood the healing that true love provides. Exactly three years after my father's death, on February 15, 2006, I gained a godson. When this happened, I knew God was smiling on me gracefully, and I embraced His love, and I was finally able to accept God's sovereignty.

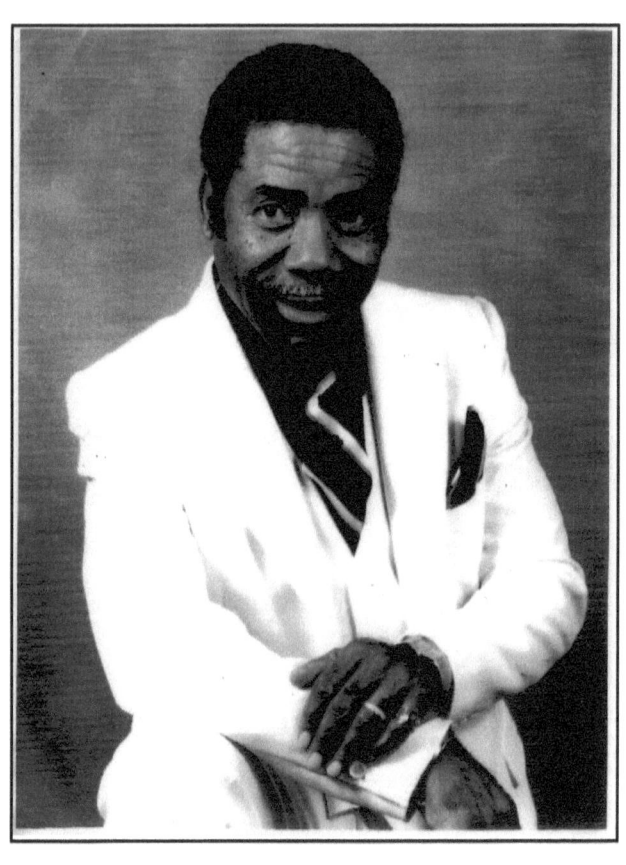

My daddy, Clyde.

I eventually sought out supportive relationships through my mom and my sister. I would journal my dreams and thoughts, which also gave me a sense of peace. I exercised, started eating better and I learned to take naps. I eventually tried new hobbies as well. I was well on my way to feeling better and living life again. Self-care was my new regime. I'd take myself to dinner and the movies. I evolved and I discovered myself again with God at the center of my healing. He made me whole and I'm grateful because months after daddy passed away, I met my best friend who became my husband, eight years later.

I could easily talk to him about what I was going through because he had lost his mom and he could understand how I felt, at times. I began to understand what was meant by God being a Wonderful Counselor, and the Prince of Peace. He spiritually arrested my mind and gave me total serenity.

Lesson: Practicing the five elements of self-care, brings clarity and revitalization to the whole person. These areas include emotional, physical, social, mental and spiritual care. Each of these are necessary for complete balance and healing.

Chapter 8

Purposed for It

Everything in our lives has a purpose, even trauma. However, traumatic situations can only build us if we refuse to allow them to control us. I remember being in second grade and writing a report on Oprah Winfrey. I admired her as a little girl. Even my teachers said I was "different" from my siblings who were all more outgoing.

The administrators and teachers at my elementary school stated that I lacked social skills. I even bit my teacher and ran away because she tried to force me to sit down and talk with her and a counselor. Nevertheless, I treated them like strangers. I was selective about who I let my guard down with. Although my parents weren't together at the time, I spent a lot of time with both of them. Not to mention, as I grew up, I experienced blatant mistreatment by a trusted relative, my mom's twin sister.

It was as if she had a hit out on my vulnerable heart. Her behavior was always chalked up as just being "mean-spirited" or it was "just her way." My aunt led me to believe something was wrong with me, too. She would say and do mean things to me and my younger brother. One time, her daughter and I got into a physical altercation, and she sided with her without asking any questions.

Many times, my brother and I would walk to and from school, and my mother's sister would drive by us as if she didn't see us. To make matters worse, to take her children to school, she had to pass by our house. Her resentment was intentional.

Even when it was freezing cold or raining, she turned her head, and blew the horn (of her 1970-something Buick) as she sped by us. The nerve! This really hurt because I thought it was something we did. I carried this pain for years, but I was constantly told to stay in a child's place, so I did.

When she stopped by our house, she was a totally different person— loving, kind and caring. What the hell?! I knew it was a front for my momma, and in my mind, she was momma's evil twin. Her wickedness caused bitterness to take root in my heart. As I got older, I chose not to connect with her, although I loved her. She looked exactly like my momma, but they were definitely two different people.

From that point on, unforgiveness was my go-to lens to quickly judge and dismiss others. My negative emotions began to metastasize like a stage

4 cancer that spread throughout other parts of my life. Ever wonder why forming meaningful relationships is hard, or trusting others is extremely difficult? We cannot purposely connect with anyone when unforgiveness has hijacked our peace and our ability to respond selflessly.

Admittedly, I only respected my aunt because she was my mom's sister. As I got older and would return home from college or the Air Force, I forced myself to go see her because my mother urged me to do so. When I visited her, I gave her gifts for birthdays, Christmas, and Mother's Day. I was certain the gifts would change her heart. I even told her I loved her, but I cannot say my words were sincere.

Finally, after several years of questioning my aunt's actions towards me, I feel resolved. This personal reconciliation did not occur because of an apology from her because she never apologized; although, her behavior changed. I reconciled my dislike towards her because God forgave me. More importantly, God revealed to me that this entire situation was never about me. However, my very existence caused her to recognize areas of her life that seemed to be unfulfilled. All of this was His way of showing me how to love people through my actions and not just words. Consequently, the love I showed her allowed me to forgive her. In 2020, God revealed that she was bitter because of her own choices and regrets.

Luke 6:31 reads: *Do unto others as you would have them do unto you.* I could clearly hear my mother say "They treated Jesus worse than others treat us, yet He died on the cross for our sins. He wants us to love in spite of." Therefore, I had to walk out Mark 11:25 in my life. How could I expect my

Father in heaven to forgive me if I did not forgive those who hurt me?

We must refuse to be the source of someone else's pain, especially a child. I had to forgive my aunt because I couldn't remain tied to all of the negative experiences for the rest of my life. Too often we become married to the pain people cause us, this keeps us stuck in the past. We cannot allow the words of others to dictate who we are. When this happens, we internalize a false narrative and as a result, we never live up to who God says we are. We are perfect and limitless in Him.

Consequently, it is through unforeseeable experiences that we discover our true identity and purpose. Ultimately, we become better than those who inflicted pain upon us. Forgiveness lets us off the hook of our own unforgiveness; not the hook of the person we may be grappling to forgive.

Lesson: We must be more than the bigger or better person. We must walk through the process, feel, heal, and forgive to become limitless. Our potential to be limitless is strategically connected to our innate ability to forgive, heal and love—it's a choice. Remember, we are purposed for it!

Chapter 9

The Limitless Formula

Throughout my life, I've been told that faith is the substance of things hoped for and the evidence of things not seen. I've also been told; all I need is faith the size of a mustard seed. I had a difficult time conceptualizing "mustard seed" faith. So, I had to see a mustard seed for myself.

As a child, my mother kept a vegetable garden, but I never paid attention to the size of any of the seeds. The garden had mustard greens, collard greens, tomatoes, peas, and corn. When momma planted her seeds, she expected a harvest. In the same manner, God expects us to be planted and rooted in Him to produce a plentiful harvest.

As a young adult, I discovered exactly how small a mustard seed is. Undoubtedly, I knew I could trust God that much (if not more). My mustard seed faith was tested when I decided to go back to school to become a nurse. This decision required me to pick up everything and move to Savannah. I trusted that God would make the necessary provisions for my life. The move was filled with several uncertainties.

During my last semester, my financial aid was delayed, and I had no idea how I'd purchase my books or fill my cupboard with needed essentials. I didn't have any extra money; I had spent it on car repairs and my mother assisted me! I had $50 to my name, if that.

At certain moments in our lives, God will allow our wells to run dry, so that we have no choice but to trust Him. I kept hearing, "Trust in the Lord with all thine heart and lean not unto thine own understanding." I felt that God was about to prove that He is Jehovah Jireh [The faithful provider]! I knew He would let me know what it meant to plant a seed (of faith) in Him and receive a harvest.

One evening, I heard a knock on my door, and I wasn't expecting company. When I opened the door, it was my friend, Prophetess Coletta. When her car broke down, I had allowed her to use my vehicle to drive mail across campus as a courier. I did it out of the kindness of my heart. I didn't want or expect anything in return.

As she walked inside, she exclaimed, "Hey Kizzy boo!" Her smile was bright and infectious! I greeted her with the same enthusiasm. Then she said, "I went grocery shopping and I picked up some things for you. You have done so much for me and other people, so I had to look out for you, too!" I wondered, "How did she know I was down to my last few meals?" Then I realized, she didn't know but God did. When we begin to trust God like never before, He will grant us unexpected blessings like *never* before.

I believe in giving to others, but it is so hard for me to receive. However, on that day, I learned it is OK to receive, especially when there's a need. Shortly after her special delivery, I remembered that my mother had given me a bag with lots of coins in it, I reserved it for tough times. I never imagined things would get that tough, but they did. So, I set aside my pride, grabbed the coins, jumped in my Honda Accord, and drove straight to Food Lion. I dumped all the coins into the machine, and to my surprise there was more than $329 in loose change and more than $100 dollars in rolled quarters! I had enough money to purchase my books, buy groceries, and I had money left over. I felt as if God had given me a personalized "two fish and five loaves" type of miracle!" Limits don't exist with God.

This is what I learned: We are not better than anyone, being judgmental is detrimental, and being sensitive to the voice of God is essential. I also realized that God knows what we need before we know. Therefore, He's already placed our needs on the heart of others. When we have faith in God's abilities [and not our own], not only will He make a way, but God will exceed our expectations in unfathomable ways.

Faith and obedience are the essential components of the limitless formula. However, obedience is another area that I struggled with until I mastered, moving by God's instruction. There were times when I allowed "self" to get in the way.

I didn't want to face another obstacle or delay in my life because of my disobedience (Deuteronomy 28:15-68). When we ignore God's instruction, we compromise more than our peace.

My past beckoned for me while I strived to reach for my future. All I wanted to do was be in the present and enjoy the gift of the day. However, I knew God had a special calling on my life. I dreamt about it repeatedly. However, I wasn't ready, because I enjoyed being "the life of the party" and didn't want to give that lifestyle up (just yet). I recall going out with my cousins to the Omega (a popular nightclub club). That was the first mistake. I thought, *God is Alpha and Omega...but it was just a club.* As I stood outside my car, I found myself eating dirt! I heard gunshots, and I knew stray bullets don't respect anybody! I'd never fallen to the ground so quickly! I knew I wasn't supposed to go, and in the back of my mind, I was fearful of the unknown. I could hear my "Auntie-mom" [my mom's youngest sister] saying, "Kizzy, you know you shouldn't be going anywhere with the name Omega in it— except church!"

One would think that would have been my last time hanging out there, but years later I visited the club again. Nothing happened this particular time, but I knew that I had outgrown that crowd. It was time for me to give God a complete yes. My life had to glorify Him, this is my ultimate purpose. I understood, if I committed my life to God, He would open unimaginable doors for me. My obedience caused an overflow of blessings, the size of my faith increased from a mustard seed to papaya seeds… papayas have numerous seeds within them and the seeds of my faith were countless.

Another component of the limitless formula is courage. I remember being so fearful to jump, not off of a ledge or anything of the sort physically. I was fearful to jump start my success, fearful of change and fearful of being the first to achieve success in my family. Fear made me comfortable with being mediocre. I was comfortable with the glass being half full and I didn't know how I would respond to winning (not to mention experiencing a winning streak). I had no desire to be in uncomfortable situations that challenged me. Then I realized that the world is full of average people but not humble and successful leaders.

Yes, I had been speaking since childhood and it came naturally, yet when the opportunity arose for me to launch out into the marketplace as a transformational speaker, I became paralyzed with thoughts of failure. Naturally, we are hard on ourselves, but I felt as if I always had to prove something to myself. It was always me versus the best me. Have you ever met someone who felt the need to one up themselves? Do you know how difficult it is to outshine yourself? Well, this is me!

Looking back, I understand the need for developing language that pushes us to becoming limitless. These are the declarations for defeating negative talk. When negative self-talk becomes our daily language, it pushes us into the direction of negative people, negative situations and a lifestyle of negativity. This also leads to blaming others without any action to change the negative narrative we replay in our lives. We are better than that and owe it to ourselves to go beyond better to limitless.

Unforgiveness, fear, depression, cycles of dysfunctional behavior, and pessimism are "coping mechanisms" of trauma; these keep us comfortable.

However, we cannot survive unexplainable situations and remain married to unproductive habits such as: negative thought patterns, poor family traits, or fear... and expect to be limitless. It is time to assess what's been limiting us!

Therefore, I had to redefine failure. If I choose not to try, that is failure. If I choose to settle, that is failure. I choose to trust in my own ability, and not God's abilities, that is failure. Thankfully, I finally understood that there is NO failure in or with God! I had an epiphany... I am limitless! NOT in my own might, but God's. He has promised me that His plans for my life WILL exceed any and everything I could possibly imagine. My imagination is quite elaborate, but more importantly my dreams, hopes, and imaginations are inspired by the promises of God.

I see what I see because God already promised I'd have it! Being limitless isn't impossible, it is necessary. So, apply the limitless formula to your life today; faith, obedience, and courage so that you will be limitless, too!

Lesson: Execute the Limitless formula: Faith + Obedience + Courage = Limitless

About the Author

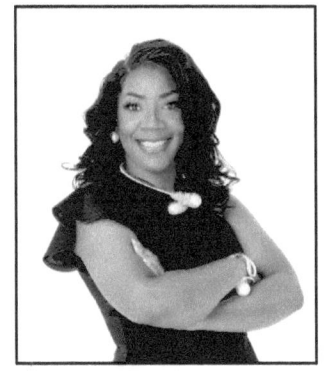

Kizzy McCray-Sheppard is the Limitless Thought Leader™, and Founder of Limitless Possibilities Now, LLC. Kizzy is a devoted woman of faith, a wife, mother, speaker, and a best-selling author. She spent some of the best years of her life serving in the United States Air Force.

Kizzy earned a Bachelor of Science in social psychology from Park University; a Bachelor of Science in nursing from Georgia Southern University at Armstrong; and a Master of Science in nursing from Chamberlain University.

After committing her life to this country, her mission continues in her work as a mentor, nurse practitioner, and entrepreneur. Her purpose is to inspire and encourage others to live out their dreams and aspirations, while focusing on self-care.

When Kizzy isn't coaching clients or keynoting events, she is enjoying quality time with her family, mini staycations, reading and trips to the spa.

For more information about Kizzy, visit: www.limitlesspossibilitiesnow.com

www.ingramcontent.com/pod-product-compliance
Lightning Source LLC
Chambersburg PA
CBHW020914080526
44589CB00011B/587